BLOOD GLUCOSE MONITORING

LOG BOOK

Records

From: _____
(date)

To: _____
(date)

Belongs to:

_____
(NAME)

BLOOD GLUCOSE MONITORING				
DAY / DATE		Breakfast	Mid - Morning	Lunch
MONDAY Date:	Glucose: Insulin/Meds:			
TUESDAY Date:	Glucose: Insulin/Meds:			
WEDNESDAY Date:	Glucose: Insulin/Meds:			
THURSDAY Date:	Glucose: Insulin/Meds:			
FRIDAY Date:	Glucose: Insulin/Meds:			
SATURDAY Date:	Glucose: Insulin/Meds:			
SUNDAY Date:	Glucose: Insulin/Meds:			
MONDAY Date:	Glucose: Insulin/Meds:			
TUESDAY Date:	Glucose: Insulin/Meds:			
WEDNESDAY Date:	Glucose: Insulin/Meds:			
THURSDAY Date:	Glucose: Insulin/Meds:			
FRIDAY Date:	Glucose: Insulin/Meds:			
SATURDAY Date:	Glucose: Insulin/Meds:			
SUNDAY Date:	Glucose: Insulin/Meds:			

BLOOD GLUCOSE MONITORING				
	Mid - Afternoon	Dinner	Nightime	Comments
Glucose: Insulin/Meds:				
Glucose: Insulin/Meds:				
Glucose: Insulin/Meds:				
Glucose: Insulin/Meds:				
Glucose: Insulin/Meds:				
Glucose: Insulin/Meds:				
Glucose: Insulin/Meds:				
Glucose: Insulin/Meds:				
Glucose: Insulin/Meds:				
Glucose: Insulin/Meds:				
Glucose: Insulin/Meds:				
Glucose: Insulin/Meds:				
Glucose: Insulin/Meds:				
Glucose: Insulin/Meds:				

BLOOD GLUCOSE MONITORING				
DAY / DATE		Breakfast	Mid - Morning	Lunch
MONDAY Date:	Glucose:			
	Insulin/Meds:			
TUESDAY Date:	Glucose:			
	Insulin/Meds:			
WEDNESDAY Date:	Glucose:			
	Insulin/Meds:			
THURSDAY Date:	Glucose:			
	Insulin/Meds:			
FRIDAY Date:	Glucose:			
	Insulin/Meds:			
SATURDAY Date:	Glucose:			
	Insulin/Meds:			
SUNDAY Date:	Glucose:			
	Insulin/Meds:			
MONDAY Date:	Glucose:			
	Insulin/Meds:			
TUESDAY Date:	Glucose:			
	Insulin/Meds:			
WEDNESDAY Date:	Glucose:			
	Insulin/Meds:			
THURSDAY Date:	Glucose:			
	Insulin/Meds:			
FRIDAY Date:	Glucose:			
	Insulin/Meds:			
SATURDAY Date:	Glucose:			
	Insulin/Meds:			
SUNDAY Date:	Glucose:			
	Insulin/Meds:			

BLOOD GLUCOSE MONITORING				
	Mid - Afternoon	Dinner	Nightime	Comments
Glucose:				
Insulin/Meds:				
Glucose:				
Insulin/Meds:				
Glucose:				
Insulin/Meds:				
Glucose:				
Insulin/Meds:				
Glucose:				
Insulin/Meds:				
Glucose:				
Insulin/Meds:				
Glucose:				
Insulin/Meds:				
Glucose:				
Insulin/Meds:				
Glucose:				
Insulin/Meds:				
Glucose:				
Insulin/Meds:				
Glucose:				
Insulin/Meds:				
Glucose:				
Insulin/Meds:				
Glucose:				
Insulin/Meds:				
Glucose:				
Insulin/Meds:				

BLOOD GLUCOSE MONITORING				
DAY / DATE		Breakfast	Mid - Morning	Lunch
MONDAY Date:	Glucose:			
	Insulin/Meds:			
TUESDAY Date:	Glucose:			
	Insulin/Meds:			
WEDNESDAY Date:	Glucose:			
	Insulin/Meds:			
THURSDAY Date:	Glucose:			
	Insulin/Meds:			
FRIDAY Date:	Glucose:			
	Insulin/Meds:			
SATURDAY Date:	Glucose:			
	Insulin/Meds:			
SUNDAY Date:	Glucose:			
	Insulin/Meds:			
MONDAY Date:	Glucose:			
	Insulin/Meds:			
TUESDAY Date:	Glucose:			
	Insulin/Meds:			
WEDNESDAY Date:	Glucose:			
	Insulin/Meds:			
THURSDAY Date:	Glucose:			
	Insulin/Meds:			
FRIDAY Date:	Glucose:			
	Insulin/Meds:			
SATURDAY Date:	Glucose:			
	Insulin/Meds:			
SUNDAY Date:	Glucose:			
	Insulin/Meds:			

BLOOD GLUCOSE MONITORING				
	Mid - Afternoon	Dinner	Nightime	Comments
Glucose:				
Insulin/Meds:				
Glucose:				
Insulin/Meds:				
Glucose:				
Insulin/Meds:				
Glucose:				
Insulin/Meds:				
Glucose:				
Insulin/Meds:				
Glucose:				
Insulin/Meds:				
Glucose:				
Insulin/Meds:				
Glucose:				
Insulin/Meds:				
Glucose:				
Insulin/Meds:				
Glucose:				
Insulin/Meds:				
Glucose:				
Insulin/Meds:				
Glucose:				
Insulin/Meds:				
Glucose:				
Insulin/Meds:				
Glucose:				
Insulin/Meds:				

BLOOD GLUCOSE MONITORING				
DAY / DATE		Breakfast	Mid - Morning	Lunch
MONDAY Date:	Glucose: Insulin/Meds:			
TUESDAY Date:	Glucose: Insulin/Meds:			
WEDNESDAY Date:	Glucose: Insulin/Meds:			
THURSDAY Date:	Glucose: Insulin/Meds:			
FRIDAY Date:	Glucose: Insulin/Meds:			
SATURDAY Date:	Glucose: Insulin/Meds:			
SUNDAY Date:	Glucose: Insulin/Meds:			
MONDAY Date:	Glucose: Insulin/Meds:			
TUESDAY Date:	Glucose: Insulin/Meds:			
WEDNESDAY Date:	Glucose: Insulin/Meds:			
THURSDAY Date:	Glucose: Insulin/Meds:			
FRIDAY Date:	Glucose: Insulin/Meds:			
SATURDAY Date:	Glucose: Insulin/Meds:			
SUNDAY Date:	Glucose: Insulin/Meds:			

BLOOD GLUCOSE MONITORING				
	Mid - Afternoon	Dinner	Nightime	Comments
Glucose:				
Insulin/Meds:				
Glucose:				
Insulin/Meds:				
Glucose:				
Insulin/Meds:				
Glucose:				
Insulin/Meds:				
Glucose:				
Insulin/Meds:				
Glucose:				
Insulin/Meds:				
Glucose:				
Insulin/Meds:				
Glucose:				
Insulin/Meds:				
Glucose:				
Insulin/Meds:				
Glucose:				
Insulin/Meds:				
Glucose:				
Insulin/Meds:				
Glucose:				
Insulin/Meds:				
Glucose:				
Insulin/Meds:				
Glucose:				
Insulin/Meds:				

BLOOD GLUCOSE MONITORING				
DAY / DATE		Breakfast	Mid - Morning	Lunch
MONDAY Date:	Glucose: Insulin/Meds:			
TUESDAY Date:	Glucose: Insulin/Meds:			
WEDNESDAY Date:	Glucose: Insulin/Meds:			
THURSDAY Date:	Glucose: Insulin/Meds:			
FRIDAY Date:	Glucose: Insulin/Meds:			
SATURDAY Date:	Glucose: Insulin/Meds:			
SUNDAY Date:	Glucose: Insulin/Meds:			
MONDAY Date:	Glucose: Insulin/Meds:			
TUESDAY Date:	Glucose: Insulin/Meds:			
WEDNESDAY Date:	Glucose: Insulin/Meds:			
THURSDAY Date:	Glucose: Insulin/Meds:			
FRIDAY Date:	Glucose: Insulin/Meds:			
SATURDAY Date:	Glucose: Insulin/Meds:			
SUNDAY Date:	Glucose: Insulin/Meds:			

BLOOD GLUCOSE MONITORING				
	Mid - Afternoon	Dinner	Nightime	Comments
Glucose:				
Insulin/Meds:				
Glucose:				
Insulin/Meds:				
Glucose:				
Insulin/Meds:				
Glucose:				
Insulin/Meds:				
Glucose:				
Insulin/Meds:				
Glucose:				
Insulin/Meds:				
Glucose:				
Insulin/Meds:				
Glucose:				
Insulin/Meds:				
Glucose:				
Insulin/Meds:				
Glucose:				
Insulin/Meds:				
Glucose:				
Insulin/Meds:				
Glucose:				
Insulin/Meds:				
Glucose:				
Insulin/Meds:				
Glucose:				
Insulin/Meds:				

BLOCD GLUCOSE MONITORING				
DAY / DATE		Breakfast	Mid - Morning	Lunch
MONDAY Date:	Glucose: Insulin/Meds:			
TUESDAY Date:	Glucose: Insulin/Meds:			
WEDNESDAY Date:	Glucose: Insulin/Meds:			
THURSDAY Date:	Glucose: Insulin/Meds:			
FRIDAY Date:	Glucose: Insulin/Meds:			
SATURDAY Date:	Glucose: Insulin/Meds:			
SUNDAY Date:	Glucose: Insulin/Meds:			
MONDAY Date:	Glucose: Insulin/Meds:			
TUESDAY Date:	Glucose: Insulin/Meds:			
WEDNESDAY Date:	Glucose: Insulin/Meds:			
THURSDAY Date:	Glucose: Insulin/Meds:			
FRIDAY Date:	Glucose: Insulin/Meds:			
SATURDAY Date:	Glucose: Insulin/Meds:			
SUNDAY Date:	Glucose: Insulin/Meds:			

BLOOD GLUCOSE MONITORING				
	Mid - Afternoon	Dinner	Nightime	Comments
Glucose:				
Insulin/Meds:				
Glucose:				
Insulin/Meds:				
Glucose:				
Insulin/Meds:				
Glucose:				
Insulin/Meds:				
Glucose:				
Insulin/Meds:				
Glucose:				
Insulin/Meds:				
Glucose:				
Insulin/Meds:				
Glucose:				
Insulin/Meds:				
Glucose:				
Insulin/Meds:				
Glucose:				
Insulin/Meds:				
Glucose:				
Insulin/Meds:				
Glucose:				
Insulin/Meds:				
Glucose:				
Insulin/Meds:				
Glucose:				
Insulin/Meds:				

BLOOD GLUCOSE MONITORING				
DAY / DATE		Breakfast	Mid - Morning	Lunch
MONDAY Date:	Glucose:			
	Insulin/Meds:			
TUESDAY Date:	Glucose:			
	Insulin/Meds:			
WEDNESDAY Date:	Glucose:			
	Insulin/Meds:			
THURSDAY Date:	Glucose:			
	Insulin/Meds:			
FRIDAY Date:	Glucose:			
	Insulin/Meds:			
SATURDAY Date:	Glucose:			
	Insulin/Meds:			
SUNDAY Date:	Glucose:			
	Insulin/Meds:			
MONDAY Date:	Glucose:			
	Insulin/Meds:			
TUESDAY Date:	Glucose:			
	Insulin/Meds:			
WEDNESDAY Date:	Glucose:			
	Insulin/Meds:			
THURSDAY Date:	Glucose:			
	Insulin/Meds:			
FRIDAY Date:	Glucose:			
	Insulin/Meds:			
SATURDAY Date:	Glucose:			
	Insulin/Meds:			
SUNDAY Date:	Glucose:			
	Insulin/Meds:			

BLOOD GLUCOSE MONITORING				
	Mid - Afternoon	Dinner	Nightime	Comments
Glucose: Insulin/Meds:				
Glucose: Insulin/Meds:				
Glucose: Insulin/Meds:				
Glucose: Insulin/Meds:				
Glucose: Insulin/Meds:				
Glucose: Insulin/Meds:				
Glucose: Insulin/Meds:				
Glucose: Insulin/Meds:				
Glucose: Insulin/Meds:				
Glucose: Insulin/Meds:				
Glucose: Insulin/Meds:				
Glucose: Insulin/Meds:				
Glucose: Insulin/Meds:				
Glucose: Insulin/Meds:				

BLOOD GLUCOSE MONITORING				
DAY / DATE		Breakfast	Mid - Morning	Lunch
MONDAY Date:	Glucose: Insulin/Meds:			
TUESDAY Date:	Glucose: Insulin/Meds:			
WEDNESDAY Date:	Glucose: Insulin/Meds:			
THURSDAY Date:	Glucose: Insulin/Meds:			
FRIDAY Date:	Glucose: Insulin/Meds:			
SATURDAY Date:	Glucose: Insulin/Meds:			
SUNDAY Date:	Glucose: Insulin/Meds:			
MONDAY Date:	Glucose: Insulin/Meds:			
TUESDAY Date:	Glucose: Insulin/Meds:			
WEDNESDAY Date:	Glucose: Insulin/Meds:			
THURSDAY Date:	Glucose: Insulin/Meds:			
FRIDAY Date:	Glucose: Insulin/Meds:			
SATURDAY Date:	Glucose: Insulin/Meds:			
SUNDAY Date:	Glucose: Insulin/Meds:			

BLOOD GLUCOSE MONITORING				
	Mid - Afternoon	Dinner	Nightime	Comments
Glucose:				
Insulin/Meds:				
Glucose:				
Insulin/Meds:				
Glucose:				
Insulin/Meds:				
Glucose:				
Insulin/Meds:				
Glucose:				
Insulin/Meds:				
Glucose:				
Insulin/Meds:				
Glucose:				
Insulin/Meds:				
Glucose:				
Insulin/Meds:				
Glucose:				
Insulin/Meds:				
Glucose:				
Insulin/Meds:				
Glucose:				
Insulin/Meds:				
Glucose:				
Insulin/Meds:				
Glucose:				
Insulin/Meds:				
Glucose:				
Insulin/Meds:				

BLOOD GLUCOSE MONITORING				
DAY / DATE		Breakfast	Mid - Morning	Lunch
MONDAY Date:	Glucose:			
	Insulin/Meds:			
TUESDAY Date:	Glucose:			
	Insulin/Meds:			
WEDNESDAY Date:	Glucose:			
	Insulin/Meds:			
THURSDAY Date:	Glucose:			
	Insulin/Meds:			
FRIDAY Date:	Glucose:			
	Insulin/Meds:			
SATURDAY Date:	Glucose:			
	Insulin/Meds:			
SUNDAY Date:	Glucose:			
	Insulin/Meds:			
MONDAY Date:	Glucose:			
	Insulin/Meds:			
TUESDAY Date:	Glucose:			
	Insulin/Meds:			
WEDNESDAY Date:	Glucose:			
	Insulin/Meds:			
THURSDAY Date:	Glucose:			
	Insulin/Meds:			
FRIDAY Date:	Glucose:			
	Insulin/Meds:			
SATURDAY Date:	Glucose:			
	Insulin/Meds:			
SUNDAY Date:	Glucose:			
	Insulin/Meds:			

BLOOD GLUCOSE MONITORING				
	Mid - Afternoon	Dinner	Nightime	Comments
Glucose:				
Insulin/Meds:				
Glucose:				
Insulin/Meds:				
Glucose:				
Insulin/Meds:				
Glucose:				
Insulin/Meds:				
Glucose:				
Insulin/Meds:				
Glucose:				
Insulin/Meds:				
Glucose:				
Insulin/Meds:				
Glucose:				
Insulin/Meds:				
Glucose:				
Insulin/Meds:				
Glucose:				
Insulin/Meds:				
Glucose:				
Insulin/Meds:				
Glucose:				
Insulin/Meds:				
Glucose:				
Insulin/Meds:				
Glucose:				
Insulin/Meds:				

BLOOD GLUCOSE MONITORING				
DAY / DATE		Breakfast	Mid - Morning	Lunch
MONDAY Date:	Glucose: Insulin/Meds:			
TUESDAY Date:	Glucose: Insulin/Meds:			
WEDNESDAY Date:	Glucose: Insulin/Meds:			
THURSDAY Date:	Glucose: Insulin/Meds:			
FRIDAY Date:	Glucose: Insulin/Meds:			
SATURDAY Date:	Glucose: Insulin/Meds:			
SUNDAY Date:	Glucose: Insulin/Meds:			
MONDAY Date:	Glucose: Insulin/Meds:			
TUESDAY Date:	Glucose: Insulin/Meds:			
WEDNESDAY Date:	Glucose: Insulin/Meds:			
THURSDAY Date:	Glucose: Insulin/Meds:			
FRIDAY Date:	Glucose: Insulin/Meds:			
SATURDAY Date:	Glucose: Insulin/Meds:			
SUNDAY Date:	Glucose: Insulin/Meds:			

BLOOD GLUCOSE MONITORING

	Mid - Afternoon	Dinner	Nightime	Comments
Glucose:				
Insulin/Meds:				
Glucose:				
Insulin/Meds:				
Glucose:				
Insulin/Meds:				
Glucose:				
Insulin/Meds:				
Glucose:				
Insulin/Meds:				
Glucose:				
Insulin/Meds:				
Glucose:				
Insulin/Meds:				
Glucose:				
Insulin/Meds:				
Glucose:				
Insulin/Meds:				
Glucose:				
Insulin/Meds:				
Glucose:				
Insulin/Meds:				
Glucose:				
Insulin/Meds:				
Glucose:				
Insulin/Meds:				
Glucose:				
Insulin/Meds:				

BLOOD GLUCOSE MONITORING				
DAY / DATE		Breakfast	Mid - Morning	Lunch
MONDAY Date:	Glucose:			
	Insulin/Meds:			
TUESDAY Date:	Glucose:			
	Insulin/Meds:			
WEDNESDAY Date:	Glucose:			
	Insulin/Meds:			
THURSDAY Date:	Glucose:			
	Insulin/Meds:			
FRIDAY Date:	Glucose:			
	Insulin/Meds:			
SATURDAY Date:	Glucose:			
	Insulin/Meds:			
SUNDAY Date:	Glucose:			
	Insulin/Meds:			
MONDAY Date:	Glucose:			
	Insulin/Meds:			
TUESDAY Date:	Glucose:			
	Insulin/Meds:			
WEDNESDAY Date:	Glucose:			
	Insulin/Meds:			
THURSDAY Date:	Glucose:			
	Insulin/Meds:			
FRIDAY Date:	Glucose:			
	Insulin/Meds:			
SATURDAY Date:	Glucose:			
	Insulin/Meds:			
SUNDAY Date:	Glucose:			
	Insulin/Meds:			

BLOOD GLUCOSE MONITORING				
	Mid - Afternoon	Dinner	Nightime	Comments
Glucose:				
Insulin/Meds:				
Glucose:				
Insulin/Meds:				
Glucose:				
Insulin/Meds:				
Glucose:				
Insulin/Meds:				
Glucose:				
Insulin/Meds:				
Glucose:				
Insulin/Meds:				
Glucose:				
Insulin/Meds:				
Glucose:				
Insulin/Meds:				
Glucose:				
Insulin/Meds:				
Glucose:				
Insulin/Meds:				
Glucose:				
Insulin/Meds:				
Glucose:				
Insulin/Meds:				
Glucose:				
Insulin/Meds:				
Glucose:				
Insulin/Meds:				

BLOOD GLUCOSE MONITORING				
DAY / DATE		Breakfast	Mid - Morning	Lunch
MONDAY Date:	Glucose: Insulin/Meds:			
TUESDAY Date:	Glucose: Insulin/Meds:			
WEDNESDAY Date:	Glucose: Insulin/Meds:			
THURSDAY Date:	Glucose: Insulin/Meds:			
FRIDAY Date:	Glucose: Insulin/Meds:			
SATURDAY Date:	Glucose: Insulin/Meds:			
SUNDAY Date:	Glucose: Insulin/Meds:			
MONDAY Date:	Glucose: Insulin/Meds:			
TUESDAY Date:	Glucose: Insulin/Meds:			
WEDNESDAY Date:	Glucose: Insulin/Meds:			
THURSDAY Date:	Glucose: Insulin/Meds:			
FRIDAY Date:	Glucose: Insulin/Meds:			
SATURDAY Date:	Glucose: Insulin/Meds:			
SUNDAY Date:	Glucose: Insulin/Meds:			

BLOOD GLUCOSE MONITORING				
	Mid - Afternoon	Dinner	Nightime	Comments
Glucose: Insulin/Meds:				
Glucose: Insulin/Meds:				
Glucose: Insulin/Meds:				
Glucose: Insulin/Meds:				
Glucose: Insulin/Meds:				
Glucose: Insulin/Meds:				
Glucose: Insulin/Meds:				
Glucose: Insulin/Meds:				
Glucose: Insulin/Meds:				
Glucose: Insulin/Meds:				
Glucose: Insulin/Meds:				
Glucose: Insulin/Meds:				
Glucose: Insulin/Meds:				
Glucose: Insulin/Meds:				

DAY / DATE		Breakfast	Mid - Morning	Lunch
BLOOD GLUCOSE MONITORING				
MONDAY Date:	Glucose: Insulin/Meds:			
TUESDAY Date:	Glucose: Insulin/Meds:			
WEDNESDAY Date:	Glucose: Insulin/Meds:			
THURSDAY Date:	Glucose: Insulin/Meds:			
FRIDAY Date:	Glucose: Insulin/Meds:			
SATURDAY Date:	Glucose: Insulin/Meds:			
SUNDAY Date:	Glucose: Insulin/Meds:			
MONDAY Date:	Glucose: Insulin/Meds:			
TUESDAY Date:	Glucose: Insulin/Meds:			
WEDNESDAY Date:	Glucose: Insulin/Meds:			
THURSDAY Date:	Glucose: Insulin/Meds:			
FRIDAY Date:	Glucose: Insulin/Meds:			
SATURDAY Date:	Glucose: Insulin/Meds:			
SUNDAY Date:	Glucose: Insulin/Meds:			

BLOOD GLUCOSE MONITORING				
	Mid - Afternoon	Dinner	Nightime	Comments
Glucose:				
Insulin/Meds:				
Glucose:				
Insulin/Meds:				
Glucose:				
Insulin/Meds:				
Glucose:				
Insulin/Meds:				
Glucose:				
Insulin/Meds:				
Glucose:				
Insulin/Meds:				
Glucose:				
Insulin/Meds:				
Glucose:				
Insulin/Meds:				
Glucose:				
Insulin/Meds:				
Glucose:				
Insulin/Meds:				
Glucose:				
Insulin/Meds:				
Glucose:				
Insulin/Meds:				
Glucose:				
Insulin/Meds:				
Glucose:				
Insulin/Meds:				

BLOCK GLUCOSE MONITORING				
DAY / DATE		Breakfast	Mid - Morning	Lunch
MONDAY Date:	Glucose:			
	Insulin/Meds:			
TUESDAY Date:	Glucose:			
	Insulin/Meds:			
WEDNESDAY Date:	Glucose:			
	Insulin/Meds:			
THURSDAY Date:	Glucose:			
	Insulin/Meds:			
FRIDAY Date:	Glucose:			
	Insulin/Meds:			
SATURDAY Date:	Glucose:			
	Insulin/Meds:			
SUNDAY Date:	Glucose:			
	Insulin/Meds:			
MONDAY Date:	Glucose:			
	Insulin/Meds:			
TUESDAY Date:	Glucose:			
	Insulin/Meds:			
WEDNESDAY Date:	Glucose:			
	Insulin/Meds:			
THURSDAY Date:	Glucose:			
	Insulin/Meds:			
FRIDAY Date:	Glucose:			
	Insulin/Meds:			
SATURDAY Date:	Glucose:			
	Insulin/Meds:			
SUNDAY Date:	Glucose:			
	Insulin/Meds:			

BLOOD GLUCOSE MONITORING				
	Mid - Afternoon	Dinner	Nightime	Comments
Glucose:				
Insulin/Meds:				
Glucose:				
Insulin/Meds:				
Glucose:				
Insulin/Meds:				
Glucose:				
Insulin/Meds:				
Glucose:				
Insulin/Meds:				
Glucose:				
Insulin/Meds:				
Glucose:				
Insulin/Meds:				
Glucose:				
Insulin/Meds:				
Glucose:				
Insulin/Meds:				
Glucose:				
Insulin/Meds:				
Glucose:				
Insulin/Meds:				
Glucose:				
Insulin/Meds:				
Glucose:				
Insulin/Meds:				
Glucose:				
Insulin/Meds:				

BLOOD GLUCOSE MONITORING				
DAY / DATE		Breakfast	Mid - Morning	Lunch
MONDAY Date:	Glucose:			
	Insulin/Meds:			
TUESDAY Date:	Glucose:			
	Insulin/Meds:			
WEDNESDAY Date:	Glucose:			
	Insulin/Meds:			
THURSDAY Date:	Glucose:			
	Insulin/Meds:			
FRIDAY Date:	Glucose:			
	Insulin/Meds:			
SATURDAY Date:	Glucose:			
	Insulin/Meds:			
SUNDAY Date:	Glucose:			
	Insulin/Meds:			
MONDAY Date:	Glucose:			
	Insulin/Meds:			
TUESDAY Date:	Glucose:			
	Insulin/Meds:			
WEDNESDAY Date:	Glucose:			
	Insulin/Meds:			
THURSDAY Date:	Glucose:			
	Insulin/Meds:			
FRIDAY Date:	Glucose:			
	Insulin/Meds:			
SATURDAY Date:	Glucose:			
	Insulin/Meds:			
SUNDAY Date:	Glucose:			
	Insulin/Meds:			

BLOOD GLUCOSE MONITORING				
	Mid - Afternoon	Dinner	Nightime	Comments
Glucose:				
Insulin/Meds:				
Glucose:				
Insulin/Meds:				
Glucose:				
Insulin/Meds:				
Glucose:				
Insulin/Meds:				
Glucose:				
Insulin/Meds:				
Glucose:				
Insulin/Meds:				
Glucose:				
Insulin/Meds:				
Glucose:				
Insulin/Meds:				
Glucose:				
Insulin/Meds:				
Glucose:				
Insulin/Meds:				
Glucose:				
Insulin/Meds:				
Glucose:				
Insulin/Meds:				
Glucose:				
Insulin/Meds:				
Glucose:				
Insulin/Meds:				

BLOOD GLUCOSE MONITORING				
DAY / DATE		Breakfast	Mid - Morning	Lunch
MONDAY Date:	Glucose:			
	Insulin/Meds:			
TUESDAY Date:	Glucose:			
	Insulin/Meds:			
WEDNESDAY Date:	Glucose:			
	Insulin/Meds:			
THURSDAY Date:	Glucose:			
	Insulin/Meds:			
FRIDAY Date:	Glucose:			
	Insulin/Meds:			
SATURDAY Date:	Glucose:			
	Insulin/Meds:			
SUNDAY Date:	Glucose:			
	Insulin/Meds:			
MONDAY Date:	Glucose:			
	Insulin/Meds:			
TUESDAY Date:	Glucose:			
	Insulin/Meds:			
WEDNESDAY Date:	Glucose:			
	Insulin/Meds:			
THURSDAY Date:	Glucose:			
	Insulin/Meds:			
FRIDAY Date:	Glucose:			
	Insulin/Meds:			
SATURDAY Date:	Glucose:			
	Insulin/Meds:			
SUNDAY Date:	Glucose:			
	Insulin/Meds:			

BLOOD GLUCOSE MONITORING				
	Mid - Afternoon	Dinner	Nightime	Comments
Glucose:				
Insulin/Meds:				
Glucose:				
Insulin/Meds:				
Glucose:				
Insulin/Meds:				
Glucose:				
Insulin/Meds:				
Glucose:				
Insulin/Meds:				
Glucose:				
Insulin/Meds:				
Glucose:				
Insulin/Meds:				
Glucose:				
Insulin/Meds:				
Glucose:				
Insulin/Meds:				
Glucose:				
Insulin/Meds:				
Glucose:				
Insulin/Meds:				
Glucose:				
Insulin/Meds:				
Glucose:				
Insulin/Meds:				
Glucose:				
Insulin/Meds:				

BLOOD GLUCOSE MONITORING				
DAY / DATE		Breakfast	Mid - Morning	Lunch
MONDAY Date:	Glucose: Insulin/Meds:			
TUESDAY Date:	Glucose: Insulin/Meds:			
WEDNESDAY Date:	Glucose: Insulin/Meds:			
THURSDAY Date:	Glucose: Insulin/Meds:			
FRIDAY Date:	Glucose: Insulin/Meds:			
SATURDAY Date:	Glucose: Insulin/Meds:			
SUNDAY Date:	Glucose: Insulin/Meds:			
MONDAY Date:	Glucose: Insulin/Meds:			
TUESDAY Date:	Glucose: Insulin/Meds:			
WEDNESDAY Date:	Glucose: Insulin/Meds:			
THURSDAY Date:	Glucose: Insulin/Meds:			
FRIDAY Date:	Glucose: Insulin/Meds:			
SATURDAY Date:	Glucose: Insulin/Meds:			
SUNDAY Date:	Glucose: Insulin/Meds:			

BLOOD GLUCOSE MONITORING				
	Mid - Afternoon	Dinner	Nightime	Comments
Glucose: Insulin/Meds:				
Glucose: Insulin/Meds:				
Glucose: Insulin/Meds:				
Glucose: Insulin/Meds:				
Glucose: Insulin/Meds:				
Glucose: Insulin/Meds:				
Glucose: Insulin/Meds:				
Glucose: Insulin/Meds:				
Glucose: Insulin/Meds:				
Glucose: Insulin/Meds:				
Glucose: Insulin/Meds:				
Glucose: Insulin/Meds:				
Glucose: Insulin/Meds:				
Glucose: Insulin/Meds:				

BLOOD GLUCOSE MONITORING				
DAY / DATE		Breakfast	Mid - Morning	Lunch
MONDAY Date:	Glucose:			
	Insulin/Meds:			
TUESDAY Date:	Glucose:			
	Insulin/Meds:			
WEDNESDAY Date:	Glucose:			
	Insulin/Meds:			
THURSDAY Date:	Glucose:			
	Insulin/Meds:			
FRIDAY Date:	Glucose:			
	Insulin/Meds:			
SATURDAY Date:	Glucose:			
	Insulin/Meds:			
SUNDAY Date:	Glucose:			
	Insulin/Meds:			
MONDAY Date:	Glucose:			
	Insulin/Meds:			
TUESDAY Date:	Glucose:			
	Insulin/Meds:			
WEDNESDAY Date:	Glucose:			
	Insulin/Meds:			
THURSDAY Date:	Glucose:			
	Insulin/Meds:			
FRIDAY Date:	Glucose:			
	Insulin/Meds:			
SATURDAY Date:	Glucose:			
	Insulin/Meds:			
SUNDAY Date:	Glucose:			
	Insulin/Meds:			

BLOOD GLUCOSE MONITORING				
	Mid - Afternoon	Dinner	Nightime	Comments
Glucose:				
Insulin/Meds:				
Glucose:				
Insulin/Meds:				
Glucose:				
Insulin/Meds:				
Glucose:				
Insulin/Meds:				
Glucose:				
Insulin/Meds:				
Glucose:				
Insulin/Meds:				
Glucose:				
Insulin/Meds:				
Glucose:				
Insulin/Meds:				
Glucose:				
Insulin/Meds:				
Glucose:				
Insulin/Meds:				
Glucose:				
Insulin/Meds:				
Glucose:				
Insulin/Meds:				
Glucose:				
Insulin/Meds:				
Glucose:				
Insulin/Meds:				

BLOOD GLUCOSE MONITORING				
DAY / DATE		Breakfast	Mid - Morning	Lunch
MONDAY Date:	Glucose: Insulin/Meds:			
TUESDAY Date:	Glucose: Insulin/Meds:			
WEDNESDAY Date:	Glucose: Insulin/Meds:			
THURSDAY Date:	Glucose: Insulin/Meds:			
FRIDAY Date:	Glucose: Insulin/Meds:			
SATURDAY Date:	Glucose: Insulin/Meds:			
SUNDAY Date:	Glucose: Insulin/Meds:			
MONDAY Date:	Glucose: Insulin/Meds:			
TUESDAY Date:	Glucose: Insulin/Meds:			
WEDNESDAY Date:	Glucose: Insulin/Meds:			
THURSDAY Date:	Glucose: Insulin/Meds:			
FRIDAY Date:	Glucose: Insulin/Meds:			
SATURDAY Date:	Glucose: Insulin/Meds:			
SUNDAY Date:	Glucose: Insulin/Meds:			

BLOOD GLUCOSE MONITORING				
	Mid - Afternoon	Dinner	Nightime	Comments
Glucose: Insulin/Meds:				
Glucose: Insulin/Meds:				
Glucose: Insulin/Meds:				
Glucose: Insulin/Meds:				
Glucose: Insulin/Meds:				
Glucose: Insulin/Meds:				
Glucose: Insulin/Meds:				
Glucose: Insulin/Meds:				
Glucose: Insulin/Meds:				
Glucose: Insulin/Meds:				
Glucose: Insulin/Meds:				
Glucose: Insulin/Meds:				
Glucose: Insulin/Meds:				
Glucose: Insulin/Meds:				

BLOOD GLUCOSE MONITORING				
DAY / DATE		Breakfast	Mid - Morning	Lunch
MONDAY Date:	Glucose:			
	Insulin/Meds:			
TUESDAY Date:	Glucose:			
	Insulin/Meds:			
WEDNESDAY Date:	Glucose:			
	Insulin/Meds:			
THURSDAY Date:	Glucose:			
	Insulin/Meds:			
FRIDAY Date:	Glucose:			
	Insulin/Meds:			
SATURDAY Date:	Glucose:			
	Insulin/Meds:			
SUNDAY Date:	Glucose:			
	Insulin/Meds:			
MONDAY Date:	Glucose:			
	Insulin/Meds:			
TUESDAY Date:	Glucose:			
	Insulin/Meds:			
WEDNESDAY Date:	Glucose:			
	Insulin/Meds:			
THURSDAY Date:	Glucose:			
	Insulin/Meds:			
FRIDAY Date:	Glucose:			
	Insulin/Meds:			
SATURDAY Date:	Glucose:			
	Insulin/Meds:			
SUNDAY Date:	Glucose:			
	Insulin/Meds:			

BLOOD GLUCOSE MONITORING				
	Mid - Afternoon	Dinner	Nightime	Comments
Glucose:				
Insulin/Meds:				
Glucose:				
Insulin/Meds:				
Glucose:				
Insulin/Meds:				
Glucose:				
Insulin/Meds:				
Glucose:				
Insulin/Meds:				
Glucose:				
Insulin/Meds:				
Glucose:				
Insulin/Meds:				
Glucose:				
Insulin/Meds:				
Glucose:				
Insulin/Meds:				
Glucose:				
Insulin/Meds:				
Glucose:				
Insulin/Meds:				
Glucose:				
Insulin/Meds:				
Glucose:				
Insulin/Meds:				
Glucose:				
Insulin/Meds:				

BLOCK GLUCOSE MONITORING				
DAY / DATE		Breakfast	Mid - Morning	Lunch
MONDAY Date:	Glucose:			
	Insulin/Meds:			
TUESDAY Date:	Glucose:			
	Insulin/Meds:			
WEDNESDAY Date:	Glucose:			
	Insulin/Meds:			
THURSDAY Date:	Glucose:			
	Insulin/Meds:			
FRIDAY Date:	Glucose:			
	Insulin/Meds:			
SATURDAY Date:	Glucose:			
	Insulin/Meds:			
SUNDAY Date:	Glucose:			
	Insulin/Meds:			
MONDAY Date:	Glucose:			
	Insulin/Meds:			
TUESDAY Date:	Glucose:			
	Insulin/Meds:			
WEDNESDAY Date:	Glucose:			
	Insulin/Meds:			
THURSDAY Date:	Glucose:			
	Insulin/Meds:			
FRIDAY Date:	Glucose:			
	Insulin/Meds:			
SATURDAY Date:	Glucose:			
	Insulin/Meds:			
SUNDAY Date:	Glucose:			
	Insulin/Meds:			

BLOOD GLUCOSE MONITORING				
	Mid - Afternoon	Dinner	Nightime	Comments
Glucose: Insulin/Meds:				
Glucose: Insulin/Meds:				
Glucose: Insulin/Meds:				
Glucose: Insulin/Meds:				
Glucose: Insulin/Meds:				
Glucose: Insulin/Meds:				
Glucose: Insulin/Meds:				
Glucose: Insulin/Meds:				
Glucose: Insulin/Meds:				
Glucose: Insulin/Meds:				
Glucose: Insulin/Meds:				
Glucose: Insulin/Meds:				
Glucose: Insulin/Meds:				
Glucose: Insulin/Meds:				

BLOOD GLUCOSE MONITORING				
DAY / DATE		Breakfast	Mid - Morning	Lunch
MONDAY Date:	Glucose: Insulin/Meds:			
TUESDAY Date:	Glucose: Insulin/Meds:			
WEDNESDAY Date:	Glucose: Insulin/Meds:			
THURSDAY Date:	Glucose: Insulin/Meds:			
FRIDAY Date:	Glucose: Insulin/Meds:			
SATURDAY Date:	Glucose: Insulin/Meds:			
SUNDAY Date:	Glucose: Insulin/Meds:			
MONDAY Date:	Glucose: Insulin/Meds:			
TUESDAY Date:	Glucose: Insulin/Meds:			
WEDNESDAY Date:	Glucose: Insulin/Meds:			
THURSDAY Date:	Glucose: Insulin/Meds:			
FRIDAY Date:	Glucose: Insulin/Meds:			
SATURDAY Date:	Glucose: Insulin/Meds:			
SUNDAY Date:	Glucose: Insulin/Meds:			

BLOOD GLUCOSE MONITORING				
	Mid - Afternoon	Dinner	Nightime	Comments
Glucose:				
Insulin/Meds:				
Glucose:				
Insulin/Meds:				
Glucose:				
Insulin/Meds:				
Glucose:				
Insulin/Meds:				
Glucose:				
Insulin/Meds:				
Glucose:				
Insulin/Meds:				
Glucose:				
Insulin/Meds:				
Glucose:				
Insulin/Meds:				
Glucose:				
Insulin/Meds:				
Glucose:				
Insulin/Meds:				
Glucose:				
Insulin/Meds:				
Glucose:				
Insulin/Meds:				
Glucose:				
Insulin/Meds:				
Glucose:				
Insulin/Meds:				

BLOCK GLUCOSE MONITORING				
DAY / DATE		Breakfast	Mid - Morning	Lunch
MONDAY Date:	Glucose:			
	Insulin/Meds:			
TUESDAY Date:	Glucose:			
	Insulin/Meds:			
WEDNESDAY Date:	Glucose:			
	Insulin/Meds:			
THURSDAY Date:	Glucose:			
	Insulin/Meds:			
FRIDAY Date:	Glucose:			
	Insulin/Meds:			
SATURDAY Date:	Glucose:			
	Insulin/Meds:			
SUNDAY Date:	Glucose:			
	Insulin/Meds:			
MONDAY Date:	Glucose:			
	Insulin/Meds:			
TUESDAY Date:	Glucose:			
	Insulin/Meds:			
WEDNESDAY Date:	Glucose:			
	Insulin/Meds:			
THURSDAY Date:	Glucose:			
	Insulin/Meds:			
FRIDAY Date:	Glucose:			
	Insulin/Meds:			
SATURDAY Date:	Glucose:			
	Insulin/Meds:			
SUNDAY Date:	Glucose:			
	Insulin/Meds:			

BLOOD GLUCOSE MONITORING				
	Mid - Afternoon	Dinner	Nightime	Comments
Glucose: Insulin/Meds:				
Glucose: Insulin/Meds:				
Glucose: Insulin/Meds:				
Glucose: Insulin/Meds:				
Glucose: Insulin/Meds:				
Glucose: Insulin/Meds:				
Glucose: Insulin/Meds:				
Glucose: Insulin/Meds:				
Glucose: Insulin/Meds:				
Glucose: Insulin/Meds:				
Glucose: Insulin/Meds:				
Glucose: Insulin/Meds:				
Glucose: Insulin/Meds:				
Glucose: Insulin/Meds:				

BLOOD GLUCOSE MONITORING				
DAY / DATE		Breakfast	Mid - Morning	Lunch
MONDAY Date:	Glucose:			
	Insulin/Meds:			
TUESDAY Date:	Glucose:			
	Insulin/Meds:			
WEDNESDAY Date:	Glucose:			
	Insulin/Meds:			
THURSDAY Date:	Glucose:			
	Insulin/Meds:			
FRIDAY Date:	Glucose:			
	Insulin/Meds:			
SATURDAY Date:	Glucose:			
	Insulin/Meds:			
SUNDAY Date:	Glucose:			
	Insulin/Meds:			
MONDAY Date:	Glucose:			
	Insulin/Meds:			
TUESDAY Date:	Glucose:			
	Insulin/Meds:			
WEDNESDAY Date:	Glucose:			
	Insulin/Meds:			
THURSDAY Date:	Glucose:			
	Insulin/Meds:			
FRIDAY Date:	Glucose:			
	Insulin/Meds:			
SATURDAY Date:	Glucose:			
	Insulin/Meds:			
SUNDAY Date:	Glucose:			
	Insulin/Meds:			

BLOOD GLUCOSE MONITORING				
	Mid - Afternoon	Dinner	Nightime	Comments
Glucose:				
Insulin/Meds:				
Glucose:				
Insulin/Meds:				
Glucose:				
Insulin/Meds:				
Glucose:				
Insulin/Meds:				
Glucose:				
Insulin/Meds:				
Glucose:				
Insulin/Meds:				
Glucose:				
Insulin/Meds:				
Glucose:				
Insulin/Meds:				
Glucose:				
Insulin/Meds:				
Glucose:				
Insulin/Meds:				
Glucose:				
Insulin/Meds:				
Glucose:				
Insulin/Meds:				
Glucose:				
Insulin/Meds:				
Glucose:				
Insulin/Meds:				

BLOOD GLUCOSE MONITORING				
DAY / DATE		Breakfast	Mid - Morning	Lunch
MONDAY Date:	Glucose: Insulin/Meds:			
TUESDAY Date:	Glucose: Insulin/Meds:			
WEDNESDAY Date:	Glucose: Insulin/Meds:			
THURSDAY Date:	Glucose: Insulin/Meds:			
FRIDAY Date:	Glucose: Insulin/Meds:			
SATURDAY Date:	Glucose: Insulin/Meds:			
SUNDAY Date:	Glucose: Insulin/Meds:			
MONDAY Date:	Glucose: Insulin/Meds:			
TUESDAY Date:	Glucose: Insulin/Meds:			
WEDNESDAY Date:	Glucose: Insulin/Meds:			
THURSDAY Date:	Glucose: Insulin/Meds:			
FRIDAY Date:	Glucose: Insulin/Meds:			
SATURDAY Date:	Glucose: Insulin/Meds:			
SUNDAY Date:	Glucose: Insulin/Meds:			

BLOOD GLUCOSE MONITORING				
	Mid - Afternoon	Dinner	Nightime	Comments
Glucose: Insulin/Meds:				
Glucose: Insulin/Meds:				
Glucose: Insulin/Meds:				
Glucose: Insulin/Meds:				
Glucose: Insulin/Meds:				
Glucose: Insulin/Meds:				
Glucose: Insulin/Meds:				
Glucose: Insulin/Meds:				
Glucose: Insulin/Meds:				
Glucose: Insulin/Meds:				
Glucose: Insulin/Meds:				
Glucose: Insulin/Meds:				
Glucose: Insulin/Meds:				
Glucose: Insulin/Meds:				

BLOOD GLUCOSE MONITORING				
DAY / DATE		Breakfast	Mid - Morning	Lunch
MONDAY Date:	Glucose: Insulin/Meds:			
TUESDAY Date:	Glucose: Insulin/Meds:			
WEDNESDAY Date:	Glucose: Insulin/Meds:			
THURSDAY Date:	Glucose: Insulin/Meds:			
FRIDAY Date:	Glucose: Insulin/Meds:			
SATURDAY Date:	Glucose: Insulin/Meds:			
SUNDAY Date:	Glucose: Insulin/Meds:			
MONDAY Date:	Glucose: Insulin/Meds:			
TUESDAY Date:	Glucose: Insulin/Meds:			
WEDNESDAY Date:	Glucose: Insulin/Meds:			
THURSDAY Date:	Glucose: Insulin/Meds:			
FRIDAY Date:	Glucose: Insulin/Meds:			
SATURDAY Date:	Glucose: Insulin/Meds:			
SUNDAY Date:	Glucose: Insulin/Meds:			

BLOOD GLUCOSE MONITORING				
	Mid - Afternoon	Dinner	Nightime	Comments
Glucose: Insulin/Meds:				
Glucose: Insulin/Meds:				
Glucose: Insulin/Meds:				
Glucose: Insulin/Meds:				
Glucose: Insulin/Meds:				
Glucose: Insulin/Meds:				
Glucose: Insulin/Meds:				
Glucose: Insulin/Meds:				
Glucose: Insulin/Meds:				
Glucose: Insulin/Meds:				
Glucose: Insulin/Meds:				
Glucose: Insulin/Meds:				
Glucose: Insulin/Meds:				
Glucose: Insulin/Meds:				

VITALS CHARTS

Date	Temp	B/P	Pulse	Oxy	Blood Glucose	Height	Weight	Initials	NOTES:

Notes:

"Patience, persistence, & perspiration make an unbeatable combination for success." Napoleon Hill

Date	Temp	B/P	Pulse	Oxy	Blood Glucose	Height	Weight	Initials	NOTES:

VITALS

Notes:

"Take care of your body. It's the only place you have to live in." Jim Rohn wishestrumpet.com

Date	VITALS								NOTES:
	Temp	B/P	Pulse	Oxy	Blood Glucose	Height	Weight	Initials	

Notes:

Date	Temp	B/P	Pulse	Oxy	Blood Glucose	Height	Weight	Initials	NOTES:

VITALS

Notes:

Date	Temp	B/P	VITALS Pulse	Oxy	Blood Glucose	Height	Weight	Initials	NOTES:

Notes:

Date	Temp	B/P	Pulse	Oxy	Blood Glucose	Height	Weight	Initials	NOTES:

VITALS

Notes:

Date	VITALS								NOTES:
	Temp	B/P	Pulse	Oxy	Blood Glucose	Height	Weight	Initials	

Notes:

Date	Temp	B/P	Pulse	Oxy	Blood Glucose	Height	Weight	Initials	NOTES:

(Columns Temp, B/P, Pulse, Oxy, Blood Glucose are grouped under **VITALS**.)

Notes:

Date	Temp	B/P	Pulse	Oxy	Blood Glucose	Height	Weight	Initials	NOTES:

VITALS

Notes:

		VITALS			Blood				NOTES:
Date	Temp	B/P	Pulse	Oxy	Glucose	Height	Weight	Initials	

Notes:

Date	Temp	B/P	VITALS Pulse	Oxy	Blood Glucose	Height	Weight	Initials	NOTES:

Notes:

Date	VITALS								NOTES:
	Temp	B/P	Pulse	Oxy	Blood Glucose	Height	Weight	Initials	

Notes:

CUSTOMIZABLE CHART
TITLE:

CUSTOMIZABLE CHART							
TITLE:							

Customizable Chart				
TITLE:				
TITLE:				

Customizable Chart

TITLE:

CUSTOMIZABLE CHART

TITLE:

CUSTOMIZABLE CHART								
TITLE:								
CUSTOMIZABLE CHART								
TITLE:								

QUESTIONS TO ASK DOCTOR AT NEXT VISIT:

DATE OF DOCTOR APPOINTMENT:

NOTES:

QUESTIONS TO ASK DOCTOR AT NEXT VISIT:

DATE OF DOCTOR APPOINTMENT:

NOTES:

QUESTIONS TO ASK DOCTOR AT NEXT VISIT:

DATE OF DOCTOR APPOINTMENT:

NOTES:

QUESTIONS TO ASK DOCTOR AT NEXT VISIT:

DATE OF DOCTOR APPOINTMENT:

NOTES:

QUESTIONS TO ASK DOCTOR AT NEXT VISIT:

DATE OF DOCTOR APPOINTMENT:

NOTES:

QUESTIONS TO ASK DOCTOR AT NEXT VISIT:

DATE OF DOCTOR APPOINTMENT:

NOTES:

NOTES:

NOTES:

NOTES:

Printed in Great Britain
by Amazon.co.uk, Ltd.,
Marston Gate.